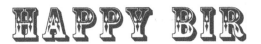

CW00497707

Love, Be...

ON YOUR SPECIAL DAY

ENJOY THE WIT AND WISDOM OF

BETTE DAVIS

FIRST LADY OF THE AMERICAN SCREEN

Edited by Jade Riley

CELEBRATION BOOKS

THIS IS A CELEBRATION BOOK

Published by Celebration Books 2023
Celebration Books is an imprint of Dean Street Press

Text & Design Copyright © 2023 Celebration Books

Cover by DSP

ISBN 978 1 915393 56 2

www.deanstreetpress.co.uk

HAPPY BIRTHDAY—LOVE, BETTE

Born in 1908 in Lowell, Massachusetts, Bette Davis knew how to make an entrance. "I happened between a clap of thunder and a streak of lightning." Despite these stormy beginnings, Bette felt from the start that she was intended for great things. Arriving in Hollywood at the age of 22, only five years later she won the Academy Award for *Dangerous*. Dangerous she was, and not afraid for a moment to play jezebels and harridans, unlikeable women and vulgar waitresses. Bette never considered herself a beauty, but we only have to look at those early films to contradict that. (Don't tell Bette!) With her curly blonde hair, those magnificent blue eyes and her tremendous screen presence, she possessed the allure of the all time greats. Early training on the stages of Broadway and those first failures in Hollywood infused Bette with the steel core she needed to make it big. Later she would be called "Mother Goddam" and La Lupe (the wolf) as she ruled Hollywood with an iron fist, without the velvet glove.

Who can blame Bette for keeping a tenacious grip on a world governed by men, accompanied by the marked competition of other talented beauties in that Golden Age of cinema? In retrospect, she need not have worried. Her successes were many; two Academy awards, ten nominations, Golden Globes, Cannes Festival Award for Best Actress, Kennedy

Center Honors and a Lifetime Achievement from the Academy, the first for a woman! Bette stated that that her greatest pride was creating the Hollywood Canteen; a support center to entertain troops returning from battle in World War II. For this she was given The Distinguished Civilian Service Medal. How very fitting for our First Lady of the American Screen.

Laugh out loud with the caustic and delightful words and wisdom of the one and only Bette Davis. And have a very Bette Birthday.

Bette Davis

There comes a time
in every woman's life
when the only thing
that helps is a glass of
champagne.

I'm the nicest goddamn dame that ever lived.

You see, I'm
an Aries.
I never lose.

Everybody
has a heart.
Except some
people.

When a man gives his opinion, he's a man. When a woman gives her opinion, she's a bitch.

If you have never
been hated by your
child, you have
never been
a parent.

It's better to be hated for who you are, than to be loved for someone you're not. It's a sign of your worth sometimes, if you're hated by the right people.

Old age ain't no place for sissies.

The key to life
is accepting
challenges. Once
someone stops doing
this, he's dead.

You should know me
well enough by now
to know I don't ask
for things I don't think
I can get.

Love is not enough. It must be the foundation, the cornerstone—but not the complete structure. It is much too pliable, too yielding.

I will not retire
while I've still got
my legs and my
makeup box.

Pleasure of love
lasts but a moment.
Pain of love lasts a
lifetime.

Home is where you go to when you've nowhere to go.

I was thought to be 'stuck up.' I wasn't. I was just sure of myself. This is and always has been an unforgivable quality to the unsure.

If everybody likes you, you're pretty dull.

You will never be
happier than you
expect. To change
your happiness, change
your expectation.

Discipline is a symbol of caring to a child. He needs guidance. If there is love, there is no such thing as being too tough with a child. A parent must also not be afraid to hang himself.

A sure way to
lose happiness, I
found, is to want it
at the expense of
everything else.

I'd love to
kiss ya but I
just washed
my hair.

I never wished I'd been a man.
I always felt like a woman and
wanted to be a woman. I wanted
to be fulfilled professionally and
personally, as a woman. There
are some who might say I had
penis envy, but I only had penis
admiration.

Brought up to respect
the conventions,
love had to end in
marriage. I'm afraid
it did.

Success only breeds a new goal.

Some young Hollywood starlets remind me of my grandmother's old farmhouse—all painted up nice on the front side, a big swing on the backside, and nothing whatsoever in the attic.

If you want a thing
done well, get
a couple of old
broads to do it.

Life is the past, the present, and the perhaps.

There may be a heaven, but if Joan Crawford is there, I'm not going.

Men become much more attractive when they start looking older. But it doesn't do much for women, though we do have an advantage: makeup.

This became a credo of mine . . . attempt the impossible in order to improve your work.

To fulfill a dream, to be
allowed to sweat over
lovely labor, to be given
the chance to create, is the
meat and potatoes of life.
The money is the gravy.

She was made up of so many things, my mother. Brutal honesty and silly deceits; self-indulgence and endless sacrifices; love and loyalty and that abundance of joy of living.

I have been
uncompromising, peppery,
intractable, monomaniacal,
tactless, volatile, and
oftentimes disagreeable . . . I
suppose I'm larger than life.

My passions were all gathered together like fingers that made a fist. Drive is considered aggression today; I knew it then as purpose.

Without discipline and detachment, an actor is an emotional slob, spilling his insides out. This abandonment is having an unfortunate vogue. It is tasteless, formless, absurd. Without containment, there is no art.

Today everyone is a star—they're all billed as 'starring' or 'also starring'. In my day, we earned that recognition.

One can make
more enemies as
a female with a
brain, I think.

Joan Crawford is a movie star. I am an actress.

It's a rare man who can stand being around an intelligent woman, let alone married to her.

It has been my experience that one cannot, in any shape or form, depend on human relations for lasting reward. It is only work that truly satisfies.

[On gay men:] Let me say, a more artistic, appreciative group of people for the arts does not exist . . . They are more knowledgeable, more loving of the arts. They make the average male look stupid.

You've got to know someone pretty well to hate them.

Among the reasons marriages fail, sex ranks no higher than fourth, behind money, having only one bathroom, and an inability to communicate, reasons one, two and three.

The best time I ever had
with Joan Crawford was
when I pushed her down
the stairs in *Whatever
Happened to Baby Jane?*

There was more good acting at Hollywood parties than ever appeared on the screen.

There's only one way to work—like hell.

You can lose
everything but
you can't lose
your talent!

The secret of
marriage is separate
bedrooms and
separate bathrooms.

Good actors I've worked
with all started out
making faces in a mirror,
and you keep making
faces all your life.

I never did pal around with actresses. Their talk usually bored me to tears.

I often think that a slightly exposed shoulder emerging from a long satin nightgown packs more sex than two naked bodies in bed.

I do not regret one professional enemy I have made. Any actor who doesn't dare to make an enemy should get out of the business.

If it doesn't
challenge you,
it won't change
you.

There is a certain
ecstasy in
wanting things
you can't get.

"

Whatever I did, I did.

"

You know what
nostalgia is, don't you?
It's basically a matter of
recalling the fun without
reliving the pain.

In this rat race
everybody's
guilty until
proven innocent.

Technicolor makes me look like death warmed over.

I have always been driven by some distant music—a battle hymn no doubt—for I have been at war from the beginning.

I became the most dedicated Girl Scout that ever lived. I would have tripped an old lady in order to pick her up.

The weak are the most treacherous of us all. They come to the strong and drain them. They are bottomless. They are insatiable. They are always parched and always bitter. They are everyone's concern and like vampires they suck our life's blood.

Your luck is how you treat people.

Temperament is something that is an integral part of the artist. Not temper, temperament. There is a vast difference.

I may not have been
wearing a mink coat, but
I was traveling with a dog.
That should have made
you think I was an actress!

I always felt special—
part of a wonderful
secret. I was
always going to be
somebody.

Strong women only marry weak men.

I survived
because I was
tougher than
anybody else.

The male ego, with
few exceptions,
is elephantine to
start with.

I'd marry again if I found a man who had fifteen million dollars, would sign over half to me, and guarantee that he'd be dead within a year.

Success is built on
disappointment,
and disappointment
is inherent in all
success.

One begins to realize
that one is getting old
when the birthday
candles weigh more
than the cake.

Being called very, very difficult is the beginning of success. Until you're called very, very difficult you're really nobody at all.

Once the love bug wears off, as it inevitably does, you are shocked to discover that you really didn't know the object of your affections at all. We know this to be so, even as we repeat the same mistake over and over and over.

I have eyes like a bullfrog, a neck like an ostrich, and long, limp hair. You just have to be good to survive with that equipment.

I am a woman
meant for a man,
but I never found
a man who could
compete.

I wouldn't piss on Joan Crawford if she were on fire.

" Pray to God and say the lines. "

I was the Marlon Brando of my generation.

Don't you hate people who drink white wine? I mean, my dear, every alcoholic in town is getting falling-down drunk on white wine. They think they aren't drunks because they only drink wine. Never, never trust anyone who asks for white wine. It means they're phonies.

She's the
original good
time who was
had by all.

People often become actresses because of something they dislike about themselves: They pretend they are someone else.

Basically, I believe the world is a jungle, and if it's not a bit of a jungle in the home, a child cannot possibly be fit to enter the outside world.

It's true we don't know
what we've got until
it's gone, but we don't
know what we've been
missing until it arrives.

I will never
be below
the title.

It is my last wish, to be buried sitting up.

I want to die
with my high
heels on, still in
action.

You know what I'm
going to have on
my gravestone?
'She did it the
hard way.'

Bette Davis

ABOUT THE EDITOR

JADE Riley is a writer whose interests include old
movies, art history, vintage fashion and books,
books, books.

Her dream is to move to London, to write like Virginia
Woolf, and to meet a man like Mr. Darcy, who owns
a vacation home in Greece.

Milton Keynes UK
Ingram Content Group UK Ltd.
UKHW011308060324
439035UK00001B/1